RUN WITH COMPLETE CONFIDENCE

The Ultimate Training Resource For Every Runner

Darryl Fry

www.advantageeducation.com.au

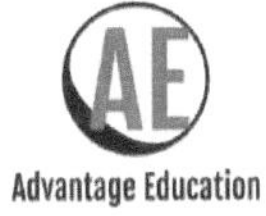

Advantage Education

CONTENTS

PRINCIPLES OF CONFIDENCE

It doesn't matter if you are a Beginning, Intermediate or Advanced runner, what you are about to read will help you to train and perform better.

You can Run With Complete Confidence because the information contained in these pages is based on principles that have been developed through years of research and practical application.

The Run with Complete Confidence Training Programs use these training principles:

- Total weekly training volume increases incrementally, allowing your body to have the best chance of absorbing and adapting to your training efforts.
- Harder sessions are generally followed by easier sessions each week.
- Easier sessions are proportional to the harder sessions in each week.
- Training programs conclude with a tapering period that varies according to the distance for which you are training.

These principles will improve your running, regardless of the distance you prefer to cover.

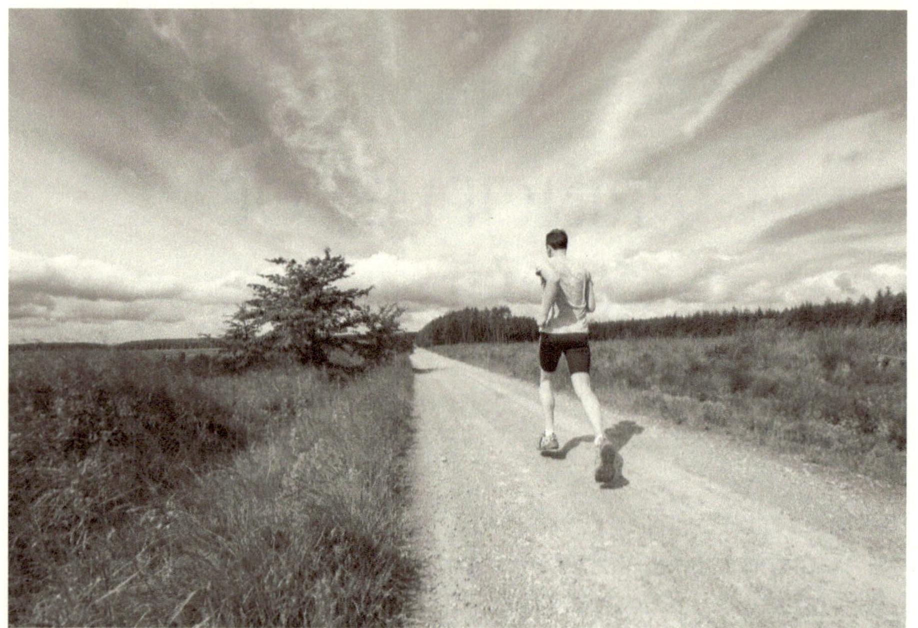

WARM UPS AND COOL DOWNS

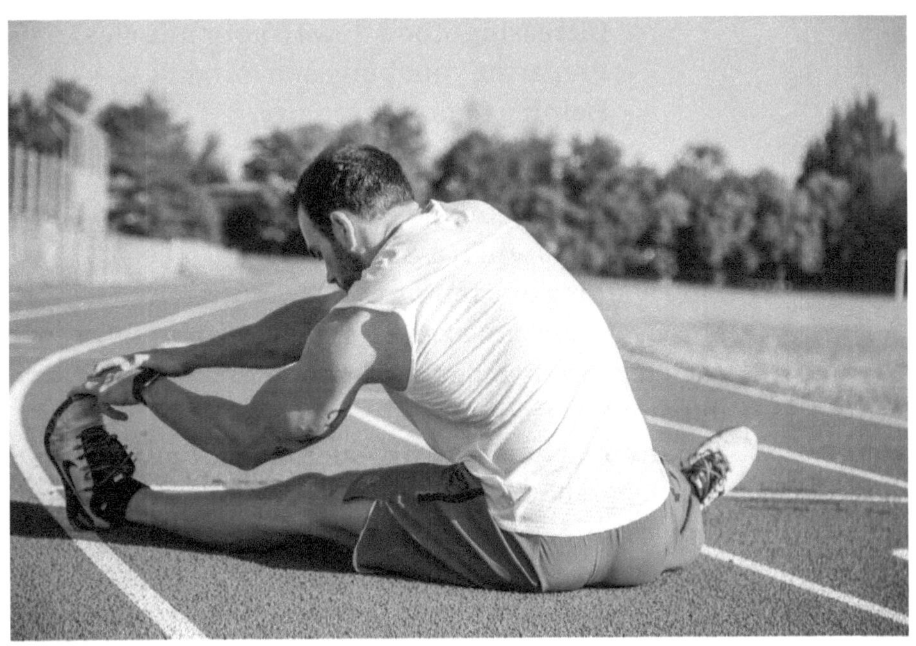

Warm Ups

Warming up is a critical part of every running session because it has many purposes. These include:

- Increasing body temperature.
- Increasing heart rate.
- Increasing blood flow to your muscles.
- Preparing your body and mind.
- Helping to prevent injury.

Your warm ups should start slowly and easily before gradually increasing in pace, complexity and intensity.

Ideally your warm ups will have four phases:

1. Easy walking or running for 8-12 minutes.
2. Muscle activation exercises such as 10 leg swings on each leg, firstly side to side, then front to back, and dynamic stretching.
3. A combination of drills such as skipping, lateral shuffle, grapevine and high knees for two minutes. Aim for three repetitions of each drill.
4. Strides over 60m-80m. Aim for four strides. Gradually progress from 60 percent of your maximum speed to about 90 percent.

Cool Downs

When you take time to cool down, you lower your heart rate more effectively and reduce the severity of post training muscle soreness.

Cool down after each run with 2-3 minutes of easy running or walking and about five minutes of low intensity static or dynamic stretching.

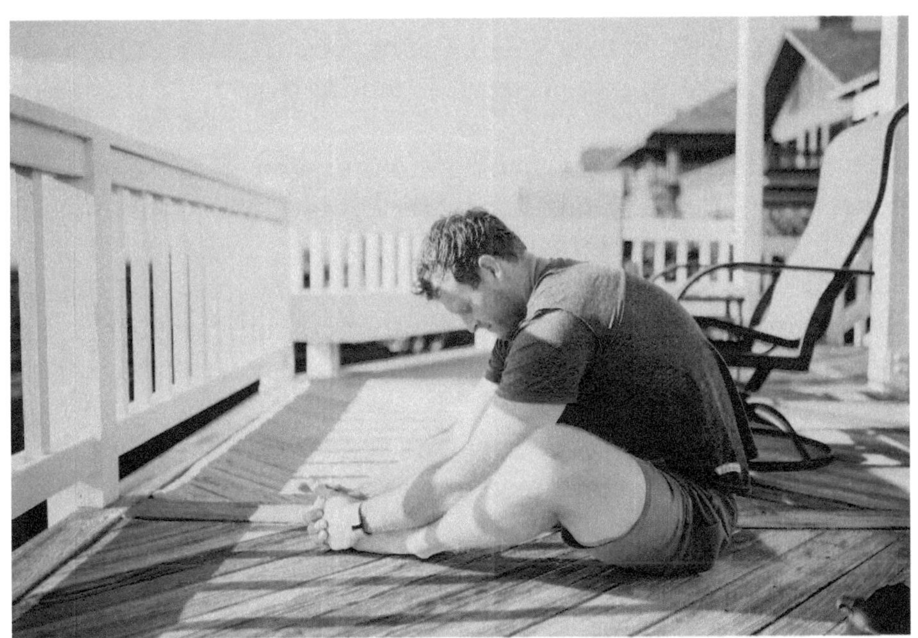

NUTRITION AND HYDRATION

Your performance will be enhanced if you complement your training by properly attending to your nutrition and hydration.

For runs lasting longer than 45 minutes, you should carry and consume an adequate supply of carbohydrate. This applies when you are training and racing.

Studies have consistently shown that consuming the proper carbohydrate sources (sugars and polymers such as glucose and maltodextrin) in the proper amounts can delay fatigue in endurance athletes.

The greatest performance benefits result when 60 to 80 grams of carbohydrate are consumed for each hour of endurance training or competition.

Sports drinks are ideal for meeting runners' nutritional needs in most training and racing situations. Sports drinks are formulated to take care of athletes' fluid, electrolyte and carbohydrate requirements and ensure that carbohydrate is delivered at the appropriate rate.

You can achieve similar results by combining energy gels with water. Energy gels have the advantage of being more portable than a drink bottle filled with sports drink. However, be aware that some energy gels do not contain electrolytes and are less easily consumed without water.

It is also worth remembering that like all athletes, you have a window of maximal opportunity for replenishing your glycogen stores. The first half hour after you finish training is the optimal time to take in carbohydrate, water and electrolytes to enhance your recovery.

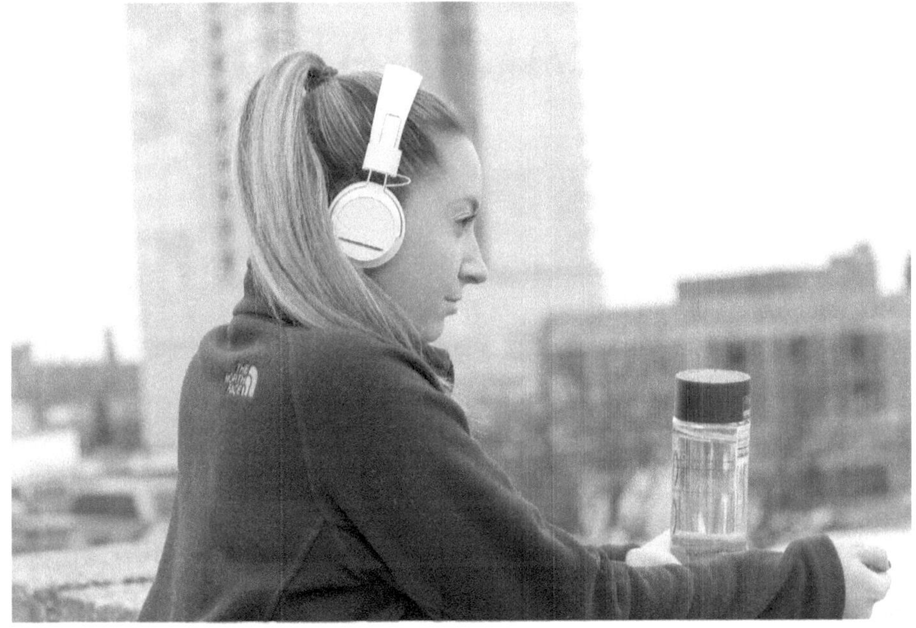

MONITORING YOUR HEART RATE

A ny device you can use to monitor your Heart Rate during your training sessions is going to give you an advantage. Research and practical experience have shown that monitoring your Heart Rate helps you to get more out of your running training.

Most wearable devices have inbuilt functions that will enable you to find your appropriate Heart Rate Training Zones.

If your device is not equipped with a feature that enables you to find your Training Zone, then use the Maffetone System of Heart Rate Training.

Dr Phil Maffetone developed his system to help endurance athletes consistently train at an appropriate intensity that uses their most important energy system, the aerobic system.

How to calculate your training zone using the Maffetone System:

1. Start with the number 180.
2. Subtract your age.
3. Take this number and correct it by the following:

- If you do not work out, subtract another five beats.
- If you work out only one or two days a week, subtract two or three beats.
- If you work out three or four times a week keep the number

where it is.

- If you work out five or six times a week keep the number where it is.
- If you work out seven or more times a week and have done so for over a year, add five beats to the number.
- If you are over about 55 years old or younger than about 25 years old, add another five beats to whatever number you now have.
- If you are about 20 years old or younger, add an additional five beats to the corrected number you now have.

The number you have now is your upper heart rate training limit in beats per minute (BPM).

Subtract ten from your upper limit to calculate your lower heart rate training limit as BPM.

Your heart rate should stay between your upper and lower heart rate training limits for the majority of most sessions.

SIZZLING SESSIONS

Sizzling Sessions are a feature of some of Run With Complete Confidence's 5km and 10km Training Programs.

Sizzling Sessions build on the principles of fartlek running training and help you to get the most out of your workout by encouraging you to adhere to specific exertion levels.

Although you can still use a device that measures your heart rate, you don't need any equipment to measure your exertion levels during a Sizzling Session. The reason for this is that your exertion levels are determined by your own perception of the effort you are putting in.

An exertion level of 10 is flat out, the hardest you can possibly go. An exertion level of 0 is at the extreme opposite end of the scale and means you wouldn't actually be moving. Most of the time during a Sizzling Session, you will be somewhere in between these two extremes.

Each Sizzling Session starts and ends with a five-minute block of activity that is an exertion level of 5. The first five-minute block is the end of your warm-up and the last five-minute block is the start of your cool down.

In between your warm-up and cool down periods are Sizzling Cycles. Each cycle consists of one minute of activity that is an exertion level of 9 or 10, followed by two minutes of activity that are an exertion level of 6 or 7.

You do as many Sizzling Cycles during your Sizzling Session as needed to get to the total time prescribed. So, if your Sizzling

Session is scheduled to be 19 minutes, then you would do three Sizzling Cycles in between your five-minute warm-up and five-minute cool down.

One of the beauties of a Sizzling Session is that you can apply it to any form of continuous activity. All you need is some sort of device to keep track of the time. If you want variety in your program or the weather is extremely inclement, you can move a Sizzling Session indoors and use exercise equipment such as a stationary bike, treadmill, stepper or elliptical machine.

5KM PROGRAMS

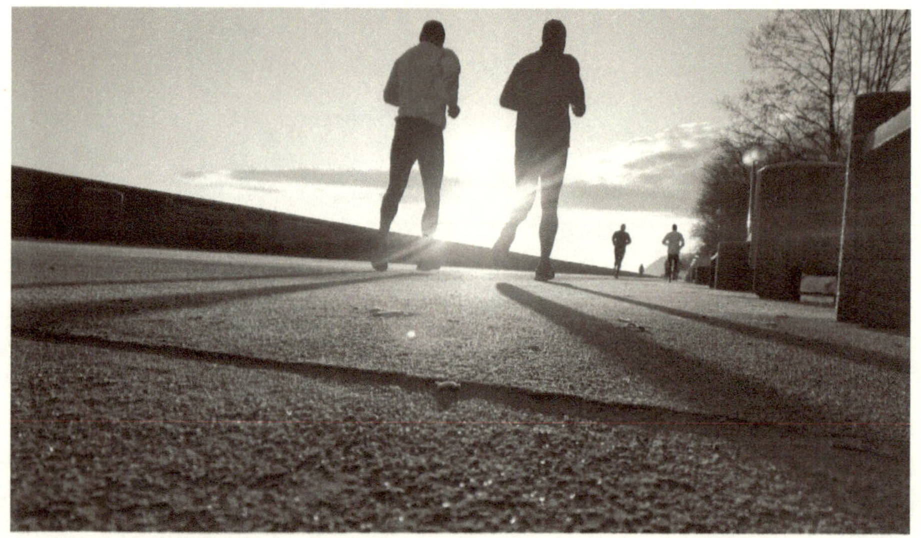

Beginner 5km Program

The Beginner Five Kilometre Program goes for six weeks and is aimed at someone who doesn't run at all yet.

There is flexibility in the program for when you do your sessions, but if possible, don't do them on consecutive days.

The Beginner Program is designed to get you to a level where you can comfortably cover five kilometres, possibly with a few short walk breaks.

It is advised that you start your five kilometre race slowly and conserve your energy. If you have followed the training program, you should be able to run at least 20 minutes before you need a walking break, but if this is not the case, don't hesitate to take a break earlier.

Week	Session					
	A	**Notes**	**B**	**Notes**	**C**	**Notes**
One	Run 1 minute, walk 1 minute. Repeat 9 times.		Run 1 minute, walk 4 minutes. Repeat 4 times.		Run 2 minutes, walk 4 minutes. Repeat 4 times.	
Two	Run 3 minutes, walk 3 minutes. Repeat 3 times.		Run 4 minutes, walk 4 minutes. Repeat 3 times.		Run 5 minutes, walk 3 minutes. Repeat 2 times.	
Three	Run 7 minutes, walk 2 minutes. Repeat 2 times.		Run 8 minutes, walk 2 minutes. Repeat 2 times.		Run 8 minutes, walk 2 minutes. Repeat 2 times.	
Four	Run 8 minutes, walk 2 minutes. Repeat 2 times.		Run 10 minutes, walk 2 minutes. Repeat and then run for 5 minutes.		Run 8 minutes, walk 2 minutes. Repeat 2 times.	
Five	Run 9 minutes, walk 1 minute. Repeat 2 times.		Run 12 minutes, walk 2 minutes. Repeat and then run for 5 minutes.		Run 8 minutes, walk 2 minutes. Repeat 2 times.	
Six	Run 15 minutes, walk 1 minute. Repeat.		Run 8 minutes, walk 2 minutes. Repeat 2 times.		Five kilometre race.	

Intermediate 5km Program

The Intermediate Five Kilometre Program goes for six weeks and is designed for anyone who can run for 30 minutes, four times a week.

If possible, the only sessions that should be done on consecutive days are Sessions C and D. Preferably these sessions should be done on the weekend.

The Intermediate Program includes Sizzling Sessions and other opportunities to vary your training pace for maximum benefit.

Week	Session							
	A	Notes	B	Notes	C	Notes	D	Notes
One	Easy run 20-25 minutes		Easy run 10 minutes Brisk run 1 minute followed by a 1 minute jog recovery. Repeat brisk run and jog recovery 3 times. Ten minute easy run.		Easy run 20 minutes.		Easy run 30 minutes.	

Week	Session							
	A	Notes	B	Notes	C	Notes	D	Notes
Two	Easy run 20-25 minutes.		Easy run 10 minutes. Brisk run 90 seconds followed by 150 second jog recovery. Repeat brisk run and jog recovery 4 times. Ten minute easy run.		Easy run 20 minutes.		Easy run 35 minutes.	

Week	Session							
	A	Notes	B	Notes	C	Notes	D	Notes
Three	Easy run 25-30 minutes		Easy run 10 minutes. Sizzling Session 19 minutes		Easy run 25 minutes		Easy run 40 minutes	
Four	Easy run 10 minutes. Time trial run for 1600 metres (1758 yards). Easy run 10 minutes.		Easy run 10 minutes. Sizzling Session 19 minutes. Easy run 10 minutes.		Easy run 20 minutes.		Easy run 45 minutes.	

Week	Session							
	A	Notes	B	Notes	C	Notes	D	Notes
Five	Easy run 25-30 minutes.		Easy run 10 minutes. Brisk run 3 minutes followed by 3 minute jog recovery. Repeat brisk run and jog recovery 2 times. Easy run 10 minutes.		Easy run 25 minutes.		Easy run 35 minutes.	
Six	Easy run 25 minutes, but include 6 x 20-40 second bursts of faster running.		Easy run 25-30 minutes.		Rest or easy run 15 minutes.		Five kilometre race.	

Advanced 5km Program

The Advanced Five Kilometre Training Program is targeted at experienced runners who can dedicate considerable time to their training.
The Advanced Program goes for 12 weeks and ideally, you should already be running 65 to 100 kilometres (40 to 60 miles) per week before starting it.

People who do this program should also have a realistic expectation that they will do their five kilometre event in a time between 17 and 20 minutes for men, or between 19 and 22 minutes for women.

Some other points to keep in mind with the Advanced Program:

•	Whenever you see 5km pace in the Advanced Program, this means the speed at which you estimate you could run a five kilometre race on that given day.

•	You should do a 1.6 kilometre (one mile) warm-up and a 1.6 kilometre (one mile) cool down before and after each fartlek session.

•	When the program refers to 4-5 hills, that means you should do four or five repeats at five-kilometre pace on a hill about 140 to 180 metres (150 to 200 yards) long.

•	Long hills should be 350 to 550 metres (400 to 600 yards) long.

•	Give yourself two minutes rest between 800 metre intervals and one minute rest between 400 metre intervals.

•	All other workouts, including the long runs, should be done at an easy training pace. A Heart Rate Monitor is ideal for ensuring you are running at an appropriate intensity.

Week	Monday	Tuesday	Wed	Thursday	Friday	Saturday	Sunday
One	Rest	6 x 800m at 5km pace	8km	10km	Fartlek 8km	6km	11km
Notes							
Two	Rest	Fartlek 8km	8km	10km	10km	6km	11km
Notes							
Three	6km	6 x 800m at 5km pace	6km	10km	6-8 hills at 5km pace	6km	12km
Notes							

Week	Monday	Tuesday	Wed	Thursday	Friday	Saturday	Sunday
Four	6km	8 x 800m at 5km pace	6km	11km	8km	6km	12km
Notes							
Five	6km	6 x 800m at 5km pace	6km	11km	6-7 long hills at 5km pace	8km	14km
Notes							
Six	6km	10 x 400m at 5km pace	6km	11km	10km	6km	16km
Notes							

Week	Monday	Tuesday	Wed	Thursday	Friday	Saturday	Sunday
Seven	6km	8 x 800m at 5km pace	6km	10km	6-7 long hills at 5km pace	6km	5km practice race or 10km easy
Notes							
Eight	6km	11km	6km	10km	6 x 400m at 5km pace minus 15 seconds per kilometre	8km	12km
Notes							
Nine	6km	10 x 400m at 5km pace	6km	11km	8-10 hills at 5km pace	6km	11km
Notes							

Week	Monday	Tuesday	Wed	Thursday	Friday	Saturday	Sunday
Ten	6km	8 x 400m at 5km pace minus 15 seconds	6km	11km	11km	6km	5km practice race or 10km easy
Notes							
11	Rest	10km	8-10 hills at 5km pace	10km	12 x 400m at 5km pace	6 km	8 km
Notes							
12	Rest	10 x 400m at 5km pace	8 km	Rest	8km	6 km	Five kilometre race
Notes							

10 KM PROGRAMS

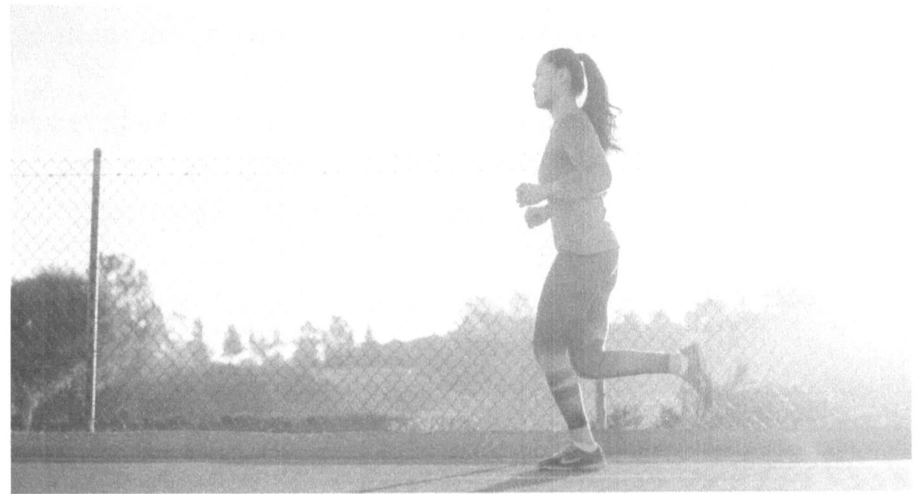

Beginner 10km Program

The Beginner Ten Kilometre Program goes for six weeks and is written for someone who is making the step up from five kilometre events.

There is flexibility in the program for when you do your sessions, but if possible, don't do them on consecutive days.

The Beginner Program is designed to get you to a level where you can comfortably cover ten kilometres in about an hour.

The program includes Sizzling Sessions and two other runs that would be best done using a Heart Rate Monitor.

When the program mentions easy runs, this refers to a pace that is about 60 to 70 percent of your maximum heart rate.

On race day, it is advised that you start slower than you think you should and gradually work your way into a comfortable, controlled pace.

Week	Session					
	A	Notes	B	Notes	C	Notes
One	Easy run 5 minutes. Sizzling Session 19 minutes.		5km		8km	
Two	Easy run 5 minutes. Sizzling Session 19 minutes.		6km		9km	
Three	Easy run 5 minutes. Sizzling Session 22 minutes.		7km		10km	
Four	Easy run 5 minutes. Sizzling Session 22 minutes.		7km		10km	
Five	Easy run 5 minutes. Sizzling Session 25 minutes.		7km		11km	
Six	5km		3km		Ten kilometre race	

Intermediate 10km Program

The Intermediate Ten Kilometre Program goes for 12 weeks and is designed for runners who are looking to take their performance to a new level.

At various stages throughout the Intermediate Program, runners will be required to cover distances that are well in excess of ten kilometres. Be aware that your longest runs during this program will build up to a peak of 16 kilometres.

Even though only three running sessions comprise the Intermediate Program, all of them are challenging and consequently should not be done on consecutive days.

Cross-training workouts, such as swimming or bike riding, can be performed on off days, but the number of these sessions should not exceed three each week.

Workout A in the Intermediate Program includes Sizzling Sessions and other opportunities to develop your speed in interval sessions.

RI in the interval sessions means Rest Interval and can be either a walk or jog recovery for the designated distance or time.

Intervals should be performed at near maximal intensity for that particular distance, but ensure you are not pushing yourself so hard that you cannot complete the full workout.

To experience the maximum benefit from workouts B and C, it is advised you use a Heart Rate Monitor.

Week	Session					
	A	Notes	B	Notes	C	Notes
One	Easy run 10 minutes. Sizzling Session 19 minutes.		1.5km warm-up. 5km HRM Training Zone. 1.5km cool down.		10km	
Two	Easy run 10 minutes. Sizzling Session 22 minutes.		1.5km warm-up. 7km HRM Training Zone. 1.5km cool down.		11km	
Three	Easy run five minutes. Sizzling Session 22 minutes.		1.5km warm-up. 6.5km HRM Training Zone. 1.5km cool down.		12.5km	

Week	Session					
	A	Notes	B	Notes	C	Notes
Four	Easy run 10 minutes. Sizzling Session 25 minutes.		1.5km warm-up. 8.5km HRM Training Zone. 1.5km cool down.		15km	
Five	15 minute warm-up. 8 x 400m with 400m RI. 10 minute cool down.		1.5km warm-up. 6.5km HRM Training Zone. 1.5km cool down.		16km	
Six	15 minute warm-up. 5 x 800m with 400m RI. 10 minute cool down.		1.5km warm-up. 8km HRM Training Zone. 1.5km cool down.		12.5 km	

Week	Session					
	A	Notes	B	Notes	C	Notes
Seven	15 minute warm-up. 8 x 400m with 400m RI. 10 minute cool down.		1.5km warm-up. 5km HRM Training Zone. 1.5km cool down.		16km	
Eight	15 minute warm-up. 4 x 1km with 400m RI. 10 minute cool down.		1.5km warm-up. 6.5km HRM Training Zone. 1.5km cool down.		12.5km	
Nine	15 minute warm-up. 4 x 1.2km with 400m RI. 10 minute cool down.		1.5km warm-up. 5km HRM Training Zone. 1.5km cool down.		16km	
10	15 minute warm-up. 3 x 1.6km with one minute RI. 10 minute cool down.		1.5km warm-up. 9.5km HRM Training Zone. 1.5km cool down.		12.5km	

Week	Session					
	A	Notes	B	Notes	C	Notes
11	Easy run 10 minutes. Sizzling Session 28 minutes.		1.5km warm-up. 5km HRM Training Zone. 1.5km cool down.		11km	
12	Easy run 10 minutes. Sizzling Session 25 minutes.		1.5km warm-up. 5km HRM Training Zone. 1.5km cool down.		Ten kilometre race	

Advanced 10km Program

The Advanced Ten Kilometre Training Program is designed for people who have previously competed in 10 kilometre events.

The advanced program goes for 12 weeks and assumes you are able to dedicate significant time to your training.

Sizzling Sessions, hill sessions and interval sessions are features of the advanced program.

Interval and hill repeats should be performed at near maximal intensity for that particular distance, but not so intensely that you cannot complete the full workout.

All other workouts should be done at an appropriate training pace measured by a Heart Rate Monitor.

RI in the interval sessions means Rest Interval and can be either a walk or jog recovery for the designated distance.

Recovery during hill repeats is when you are walking or jogging back down the hill.

Week	Monday	Tuesday	Wed	Thurs	Friday	Sat	Sunday
One	5km	Rest	8km	8km	Rest	5km	9.5km
Notes							
Two	5km	Sizzling Session 25 minutes.	8km	4 x 800m (400m RI)	Rest	5km	9.5km
Notes							
Three	6.5km	6 x Hills 60 seconds each.	8km	3 x 1km (400m RI)	Rest	6.5 km	11km
Notes							
Four	6.5km	Rest	8km	6.5km	Rest	20 minute jog.	5km time trial.
Notes							

Week	Monday	Tuesday	Wed	Thurs	Friday	Sat	Sunday
Five	6.5km	5 x Hills 90 seconds each.	9.5km	8 x 400m (200m RI)	Rest	6.5km	13km
Notes							
Six	6.5km	Sizzling Session 31 minutes.	8km	4x 1km (500m RI)	Rest	6.5km	14.5km
Notes							
Seven	6.5km	6 x Hills 120 seconds each.	9.5km	Sizzling Session 31 minutes.	Rest	8km	16km
Notes							
Eight	8km	Rest	9.5km	6.5km	Rest	5km	10km time trial.
Notes							

Week	Monday	Tuesday	Wed	Thurs	Friday	Sat	Sunday
Nine	6.5km	7 x Hills 60 seconds each.	9.5km	6 x 800m (400m RI)	Rest	8km	17.5km
Notes							
Ten	5km	Sizzling Session 34 minutes.	11km	5 x 1km (400m)	Rest	6.5km	16km
Notes							

Week	Monday	Tuesday	Wed	Thurs	Friday	Sat	Sunday
11	5km	4 x Hills 120 seconds each.	8km	8 x 400m (200m RI)	Rest	8km	13km
Notes							
12	5km	1.5km easy, 5km at race pace, 1.5km easy.	Rest	8km	Rest	20 minute jog.	Ten kilometre race.
Notes							

HALF MARATHON PROGRAMS

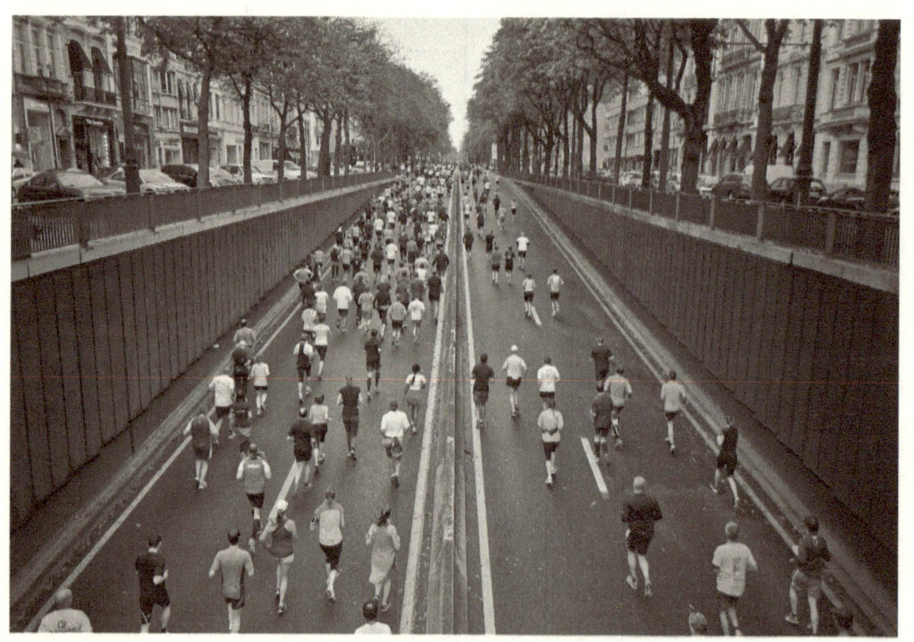

Beginner Half Marathon Program

The Beginner Half Marathon Program goes for 12 weeks and is written for someone who has previously run ten kilometre races and is now looking for a new challenge.

There is flexibility in the program for when you do your sessions, but if possible, don't do them on consecutive days.

The Beginner Program includes Sizzling Sessions and workouts that require you to stay in your Heart Rate Training Zone.

Week	Session					
	A	Notes	B	Notes	C	Notes
One	5km		6.5km		6.5km	
Two	5km		6.5km		8km	
Three	5.5km		8km		9.5km	
Four	5.5km		Easy run 5 minutes. Sizzling Session 22 minutes.		11km	
Five	6.5km		Easy run 5 minutes. Sizzling Session 25 minutes.		13km	

Week	Session A	Notes	Session B	Notes	Session C	Notes
Six	6.5km		Easy run 5 minutes. Sizzling Session 28 minutes.		14.5km	
Seven	6.5km		Easy run 5 minutes. Sizzling Session 31 minutes.		16km	
Eight	7km		Easy run 5 minutes. Sizzling Session 25 minutes.		13km	
Nine	8km		Easy run 5 minutes. Sizzling Session 28 minutes.		16km	
10	7km		Easy run 5 minutes. Sizzling Session 31 minutes.		19km	
11	6.5km		Easy run 5 minutes. Sizzling Session 22 minutes.		11km	
12	Sizzling Session 19 minutes.		20 minutes easy.		Half Marathon race.	

Intermediate Half Marathon Program

The Intermediate Half Marathon Program goes for 18 weeks and incorporates three running sessions each week.

Like the Beginner Half Marathon Program, there is flexibility within the Intermediate program for when you do your sessions. However, if possible, don't do the sessions on consecutive days.

The Intermediate Program includes interval workouts and Sizzling Sessions.

Interval repeats should be performed at near maximal intensity for that particular distance, but not so intensely that you cannot complete the full workout.

RI in the interval sessions means Rest Interval, which can be either a walk or jog recovery for the designated distance.

All other workouts should be done at an appropriate training pace measured by a Heart Rate Monitor.

If you wish to complement your training with cross training activities, such as swimming or riding, this is allowable on non-running days. It is advised you limit your cross training sessions to a maximum of two each week.

Week	Session					
	A	Notes	B	Notes	C	Notes
One	Easy run 10 minutes. Sizzling Session 22 minutes.		3.5km warm-up. 5km HRM Training Zone. 1.5km cool down.		13km	
Two	Easy run 10 minutes. Sizzling Session 25 minutes.		8km		15km	
Three	Easy run 10 minutes. Sizzling Session 28 minutes.		3.5km warm-up. 5km HRM Training Zone. 1.5km cool down.		16km	
Four	Easy run 10 minutes. Sizzling Session 22 minutes.		8km		15km	
Five	15 minute warm-up. 5 x 1km with 400m RI. 10 minute cool down.		1.5km warm-up. 5km HRM Training Zone. 1.5km cool down.		15km	

Week	Session					
	A	Notes	B	Notes	C	Notes
Six	15 minute warm-up. 3 x 1600m with 1 minute RI. 10 minute cool down.		10km		18km	
Seven	15 minute warm-up. 2 x 1200m with 1 minute RI. 4 x 800m with 2 minute RI. 10 minute cool down.		1.5km warm-up. 3.5km HRM Training Zone. 1.5km easy. 3.5km HRM Training Zone. 1.5km cool down.		16km	
Eight	Easy run 5 minutes. Sizzling Session 25 minutes.		8km		20km	
Nine	15 minute warm-up. 6 x 400m with 90 second RI. Repeat 6 x 400m with 90 second RI after 150 second break. 10 minute cool down.		1.5km warm-up. 3.5km HRM Training Zone. 1.5km easy. 3.5km HRM Training Zone. 1.5km cool down.		13km	

Week	Session					
	A	Notes	B	Notes	C	Notes
Ten	15 minute warm-up. 1.5km with 400m RI. 3.5km with 800m RI. 2 x 800m with 400m RI. 10 minute cool down.		8km		21km	
11	15 minute warm-up. 2 x 1.2km with 2 minute RI. Repeat 2 x 1.2km with 2 minute RI 2 more times after 4 minute break between sets. 10 minute cool down.		10km		16km	

Week	Session					
	A	Notes	B	Notes	C	Notes
12	Easy run 10 minutes. Sizzling Session 28 minutes.		8km		22.5km	
13	15 minute warm-up. 2 x 1.6km with 400m RI. 10 minute cool down.		10km		16km	
14	15 minute warm-up. 10 x 400m with 400m RI. 10 minute cool down.		8km		24km	
15	15 minute warm-up. 3 x 2km with 400m RI. 10 minute cool down.		1.5km warm-up. 3.5km HRM Training Zone. 1.5km easy. 3.5km HRM Training Zone. 1.5km cool down.		16km	

Week	Session					
	A	Notes	B	Notes	C	Notes
16	Easy run 5 minutes. Sizzling Session 25 minutes.		8km		20km	
17	15 minute warm-up. 5 x 1km with 400m RI. 10 minute cool down.		3.5km warm-up. 5km HRM Training Zone. 1.5km cool down.		13km	
18	Easy run 5 minutes. Sizzling Session 19 minutes.		5km		Half Marathon race.	

Advanced Half Marathon Program

The Advanced Half Marathon Training Program is targeted at competitive runners who want to improve their personal best.

The Advanced Program goes for 12 weeks and requires you to run every day of the week.

Some points to keep in mind with the Advanced Program:

• You should do a 1.6 kilometre (one mile) warm-up and a 1.6 kilometre (one mile) cool down before and after each interval and hills session.

• When the program refers to Hills, you should do repeats on a hill about 140 to 180 metres (150 to 200 yards) long.

• Long Hills workouts should be 350 to 550 metres (400 to 600 yards) long.

• Recover from hill repeats by walking or jogging back to your starting point.

• RI in the interval sessions means Rest Interval and can be either a walk or jog recovery for the designated distance.

• Interval and hill repeats should be performed at near maximal intensity for that particular distance, but not so intensely that you cannot complete the full workout.

• All other workouts, including the long runs, should be done at an easy training pace. A Heart Rate Monitor is ideal for ensuring you are running at an appropriate intensity.

Week	Monday	Tuesday	Wed	Thursday	Friday	Saturday	Sunday
One	9.5km	3 x 1500m with 2 minute RI.	6km	13km	9.5km	6.5km	19km
Notes							
Two	6.5km	6 x 800m with 2 minute RI.	8km	13km	8 x Hills	6.5km	13km
Notes							
Three	9.5km	4 x 1.5km with 2 minute RI.	8km	13km	9.5km	6.5 km	21km
Notes							
Four	6.5km	6 x 800m with 400m RI.	8km	13km	7 x Long Hills	6.5km	14.5km
Notes							

Week	Monday	Tuesday	Wed	Thursday	Friday	Saturday	Sunday
Five	9.5km	5 x 1.5km with 2 minute RI.	8km	13km	13km	6.5km	22.5km
Notes							
Six	6.5km	6 x 400m with 400m RI.	8km	16km	9 x Hills	6.5km	16km
Notes							
Seven	9.5km	6 x 1.6km with 2 minute RI.	8km	19km	9.5km	6.5km	24km
Notes							
Eight	6.5km	9 x 400m with 400m RI.	9.5km	13km	8 x Long Hills	8km	19km
Notes							

Week	Monday	Tuesday	Wed	Thursday	Friday	Saturday	Sunday
Nine	9.5km	6 x 1.5km with 2 minute RI.	9.5km	19km	9.5km	6.5km	10km race or 25.5km in HRM Training Zone.
Notes							
Ten	6.5km	10 x 400m with 400m RI.	9.5km	13km	9 x Hills	8km	25.5km
Notes							
11	9.5km	13km	9.5km	19km	13km	6.5	16km
Notes							
12	6.5km	9.5km	9.5km	13km	9.5km	4.5km	Half Marathon race.
Notes							

MARATHON PROGRAMS

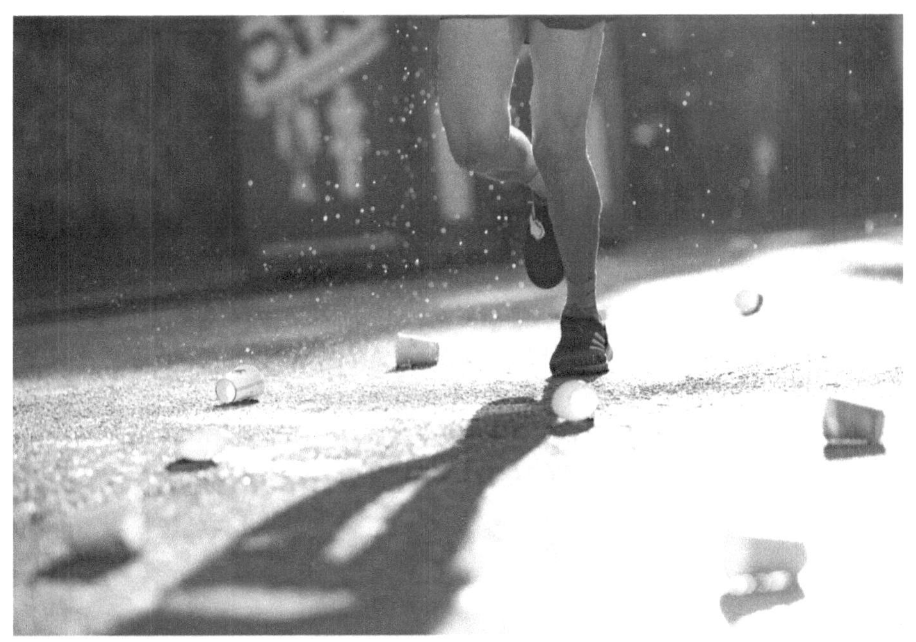

Beginner Marathon Program

The Beginner Marathon Training Program is written for someone who has previously run shorter distance races and is now looking for a new challenge.

There is flexibility in the Beginner Program for when you do your sessions, but if possible, don't do them on consecutive days.

The program includes interval sessions that should be performed at near maximal intensity for that particular distance. However, your effort should not be so intense that you cannot complete the full workout.

RI in the interval sessions stands for Rest Interval, which can either be a walk or jog for the specified distance or time.

Unless otherwise specified, all other workouts should be completed at a pace that enables you to stay in your Heart Rate Monitor Training Zone.

If you wish to complement your training with cross training activities, such as swimming or riding, this is allowable on non-running days.

Week	Session					
	A	Notes	B	Notes	C	Notes
One	15 minute warm-up. 3 x 1.6km with 1 minute RI. 10 minute cool down.		3km warm-up. 3km HRM Training Zone. 3km cool down.		13km	
Two	1.6km warm-up. 4 x 800m with 2 minute RI. 10 minute cool down.		1.5km warm-up. 8km HRM Training Zone. 1.5km cool down.		15km	
Three	15 minute warm-up. 1.2km, 1km, 800m, 600m, 400m, 200m with 200m RI. 10 minute cool down.		1.5km warm-up. 8km HRM Training Zone. 1.5km cool down.		16km	
Four	15 minute warm-up. 5 x 1km with 400m RI. 10 minute cool down.		1.5km warm-up. 8km HRM Training Zone. 1.5km cool down.		17km	

Week	Session					
	A	Notes	B	Notes	C	Notes
Five	15 minute warm-up. 3 x 1.6km with 1 minute RI. 10 minute cool down.		3km warm-up. 5km HRM Training Zone. 2km cool down.		20km	
Six	15 minute warm-up. 2 x 1200m with 2 minute RI. 4 x 800m with two minute RI. 10 minute cool down.		8km at race pace.		22km	
Seven	15 minute warm-up. 6 x 800m with 90 second RI. 10 minute cool down.		1.5km warm-up. 10km HRM Training Zone. 1.5km cool down.		25km	
Eight	15 minute warm-up. 6 x 400m with 90 second RI. Repeat above after 150 second break. 10 minute cool down.		3km warm-up. 5km HRM Training Zone. 2km cool down.		18km	

Week	Session					
	A	Notes	B	Notes	C	Notes
Nine	15 minute warm-up. 1600m (400m RI). 3200m (800m RI). 2 x 800m (400m RI). 10 minute cool down.		1.5km warm-up. 7km HRM Training Zone. 1.5km cool down.		25km	
Ten	15 minute warm-up. 2 x 1.2km with 2 minute RI. Repeat 2 x 1.2km with 2 minute RI 2 more times after 4 minute break between sets. 10 minute cool down.		16km at race pace.		20km	
11	15 minute warm-up. 1km, 2km, 1km, 1km. (400m RI between each distance). 10 minute cool down.		2km warm-up. 8km at race pace.		30km	

Week	Session					
	A	Notes	B	Notes	C	Notes
12	15 minute warm-up. 3 x 1.6km with 400m RI. 10 minute cool down.		16km at race pace.		20km	
13	15 minute warm-up. 10 x 400m with 400m RI. 10 minute cool down.		13km at race pace.		32km	
14	15 minute warm-up. 8 x 800m with 90 second RI. 10 minute cool down.		8km at race pace.		20km	
15	15 minute warm-up. 5 x 1km with 400m RI. 10 minute cool down.		3km warm-up. 5km HRM Training Zone. 2km cool down.		16km	
16	15 minute warm-up. 6 x 400m with 400m RI. 10 minute cool down.		5km at race pace.		Marathon race.	

Intermediate Marathon Training Program

The Intermediate Marathon Program also goes for 16 weeks and builds on the Beginner Program by increasing the volume of total distance in Session C.

Like the Beginner Marathon Program, there is flexibility within the Intermediate program for when you do your three weekly sessions. However, if possible, don't do the sessions on consecutive days.

The program includes interval sessions that should be performed at near maximal intensity for that particular distance. However, your effort should not be so intense that you cannot complete the full workout.

RI in the interval sessions stands for Rest Interval, which can either be a walk or jog for the specified distance or time.

Unless stated differently, all other workouts should be completed at a pace that enables you to stay in your Heart Rate Training Zone.

If you wish to complement your training with cross training activities, such as swimming or riding, this is allowable on non-running days.

Week	Session					
	A	Notes	B	Notes	C	Notes
One	15 minute warm-up. 3 x 1.6km with 1 minute RI. 10 minute cool down.		3km warm-up. 3km HRM Training Zone. 3km cool down.		21km	
Two	1.6km warm-up. 4 x 800m with 2 minute RI. 10 minute cool down.		1.5km warm-up. 8km HRM Training Zone. 1.5km cool down.		24km	
Three	15 minute warm-up. 1.2km, 1km, 800m, 600m, 400m, 200m with 200m RI. 10 minute cool down.		1.5km warm-up. 8km HRM Training Zone. 1.5km cool down.		27km	
Four	15 minute warm-up. 5 x 1km with 400m RI. 10 minute cool down.		1.5km warm-up. 8km HRM Training Zone. 1.5km cool down.		32km	

Week	Session					
	A	Notes	B	Notes	C	Notes
Five	15 minute warm-up. 3 x 1600m with 1 minute RI. 10 minute cool down.		3km warm-up. 5km HRM Training Zone. 2km cool down.		29km	
Six	15 minute warm-up. 2 x 1.2km with 2 minute RI. 4 x 800m with 2 minute RI. 10 minute cool down.		8km at race pace.		32km	
Seven	15 minute warm-up. 6 x 800m with 90 second RI. 10 minute cool down.		1.5km warm-up. 10km HRM Training Zone. 1.5km cool down.		21km	
Eight	15 minute warm-up. 6 x 400m with 90 second RI. Repeat 6 x 400m with 90 second RI after 150 second break. 10 minute cool down.		3km warm-up. 5km HRM Training Zone. 2km cool down.		29km	

Week	Session					
	A	Notes	B	Notes	C	Notes
Nine	15 minute warm-up. 1600m with 400m RI. 3200m with 800m RI. 2 x 800m with 400m RI. 10 minute cool down.		1.5km warm-up. 7km HRM Training Zone. 1.5km cool down.		32km	
Ten	15 minute warm-up. 2 x 1.2km with 2 minute RI. Repeat 2 x 1.2km with 2 minute RI 2 more times after 4 minute break between sets. 10 minute cool down.		16km at race pace.		24km	
11	15 minute warm-up. 1km, 2km, 1km, 1km, all with 400m RI. 10 minute cool down.		2km easy. 8km at race pace.		32km	

Week	Session					
	A	Notes	B	Notes	C	Notes
12	15 minute warm-up. 3 x 1.6km with 400m RI. 10 minute cool down.		16km at race pace.		24km	
13	15 minute warm-up. 10 x 400m with 400m RI. 10 minute cool down.		13km at race pace		32km	
14	15 minute warm-up. 8 x 800m with 90 second RI. 10 minute cool down.		8km at race pace.		21km at race pace.	
15	15 minute warm-up. 5 x 1km with 400m RI. 10 minute cool down.		3km warm-up. 5km HRM Training Zone. 2km cool down.		16km at race pace.	
16	15 minute warm-up. 6 x 400m with 400m RI. 10 minute cool down.		5km at race pace.		Marathon race.	

Advanced Marathon Training Program

The Advanced Marathon Training Program is targeted at competitive runners who have several marathon finishes already under their belt.

The Advanced Program goes for 26 weeks and requires you to run nearly every day of the week, sometimes twice a day, during that time.

Some points to keep in mind with the Advanced Program:

• You should start this program after two weeks rest or two weeks active rest, which can be walking or low intensity cross training.

• When the program refers to Hills, you should do repeats up a hill that takes about two minutes each time, while working between 77-90 percent of your maximum effort.

• Recover from hill repeats by walking or jogging back to your starting point.

• RI in the interval sessions means Rest Interval and can be either a walk or jog recovery for the designated distance or time.

• Interval repeats that are 1.2 kilometres or less should be performed at 85-95 percent of your maximum intensity for that particular distance.

• Longer intervals should be performed at 77-90 percent of your maximum intensity for that particular distance.

• Unless otherwise indicated, all other workouts, including the long runs, should be done at an easy training pace.

• A Heart Rate Monitor is ideal for ensuring you are running at an appropriate intensity during each session.

• Active rest refers to low intensity exercise such as walking or very easy short distance running.

Week	Monday	Tuesday	Wed	Thursday	Friday	Saturday	Sunday
One	AM and PM sessions. 6.5km each time.	13km	10km	13km	AM and PM sessions. 6.5km each time.	19km	13km
Notes							
Two	AM and PM sessions. 6.5km each time.	16km	13km	16km	AM and PM sessions. 6.5km each time.	22km	13km
Notes							
Three	AM and PM sessions. 6.5km each time.	16km	13km	16km	AM and PM sessions. 6.5km each time.	26km	13km
Notes							

Week	Monday	Tuesday	Wed	Thursday	Friday	Saturday	Sunday
Four	AM and PM sessions. 6.5km each time.	13km	10km	13km	AM and PM sessions. 6.5km each time.	19km	Rest
Notes							
Five	AM 6.5km PM 10km	16km	13km	16km	AM 6.5km PM 10km	26km	13km
Notes							
Six	AM 6.5km PM 10km	19km	13km	19km	AM 6.5km PM 10km	29km	13km
Notes							
Seven	AM 6.5km PM 10km	19km	13km	19km	AM 6.5km PM 10km	32km	13km
Notes							

Week	Monday	Tuesday	Wed	Thursday	Friday	Saturday	Sunday
Eight	AM and PM sessions. 6.5km each time.	13km	10km	13km	AM and PM sessions. 6.5km each time.	19km	Rest
Notes							
Nine	AM 6.5km PM 10km	20.5km	13km	20.5km	AM 6.5km PM 10km	32km	13km
Notes							
Ten	AM 6.5km PM 10km	20.5km	13km	20.5km	AM 6.5km PM 10km	29km	13km
Notes							
11	AM 6.5km PM 10km	20.5km	13km	20.5km	AM 6.5km PM 10km	32km	13km
Notes							

Week	Monday	Tuesday	Wed	Thursday	Friday	Saturday	Sunday
12	AM 6.5km PM 10km	13km	10km	13km	AM 6.5km PM 10km	19km	Rest
Notes							
13	AM 6.5km PM 10km	Warm up 5km. 4 x 1.6km with 3 minute RI. Cool down 5km.	20.5km	13km	Warm up 5km. 8 x Hills. Cool down 5km	32km	13km
Notes							
14	AM 6.5km PM 10km	Warm up 15 minutes. 12 x 400m with 200m RI.	20.5km	13km	AM 6.5km PM 10km	29km at Marathon pace.	13km
Notes							

Week	Monday	Tuesday	Wed	Thursday	Friday	Saturday	Sunday
15	AM 6.5km PM 10km	Warm up 15 minutes. 15 x 200m with 200m RI.	16km	13km	10km	10km race.	16km
Notes							
16	AM 6.5km PM 10km	20.5km	13km	Warm up 5km. 8 x Hills. Cool down 5km.	AM 6.5km PM 10km	32km	13km
Notes							
17	AM 6.5km PM 10km	Warm up 15 minutes. 6 x 800m with 400m RI.	20.5km	13km	AM 6.5km PM 10km	30.5km at Marathon pace.	13km
Notes							

Week	Monday	Tuesday	Wed	Thursday	Friday	Saturday	Sunday
18	AM 6.5km PM 10km	Warm up 15 minutes. 15 x 200m with 200m RI.	16km	13km	10km	Half Marathon race.	16km
Notes							
19	10km	16km	13km	Warm up 5km. 8 x Hills. Cool down 5km.	AM 6.5km PM 10km	32km	13km
Notes							
20	AM 6.5km PM 10km	Warm up 15 minutes. 4 x 1200m with 400m RI.	20.5km	13km	AM 6.5km PM 10km	33.5km at Marathon pace.	13km
Notes							

Week	Monday	Tuesday	Wed	Thursday	Friday	Saturday	Sunday
21	10km	15 minute warm-up. 15 x 200m with 200m RI.	16km	13km	6.5km	5km race.	16km
Notes							
22	10km	20.5km	13km	Warm up 5km. 4 x 1.6km with three minute RI. Cool down 5km.	10km	32km	6.5km
Notes							
23	Rest	15 minute warm-up. 15 x 300m with 100m RI.	10km	15 minute warm-up. 6 x 800m with 400m RI.	Rest	19km	Rest

Week	Monday	Tuesday	Wed	Thursday	Friday	Saturday	Sunday
Notes							
24	6.5km	Rest	15 minute warm-up. 3 x 200m with 200m RI. 400m easy. 3 x 800m with 400m RI.	Rest	8km	0-5km	Marathon race.
Notes							
25	Rest	Rest	Rest	Rest	Rest	Rest	Rest
Notes							
26	Active rest	Active rest	Active rest	Active rest	Active rest	Active rest	Active rest
Notes							

DISCLAIMER

Neither the author, nor anyone associated with the author, will be responsible or liable for any injury, accident or illness while following the programs in this book.

Always consult a medical professional before starting any exercise program.

PHOTO CREDITS

The author has sourced images for this publication from the website, Unsplash.

BOOKS IN THIS SERIES

Run With Confidence

It doesn't matter if you are a Beginning, Intermediate or Advanced runner, these books will help you to train and perform better.

All of the books in the Run With Confidence series contain information that is based on training principles that have been developed through years of research and practical application by the author.

Run 5Km With Confidence

Run 10Km With Confidence

Run A Half Marathon With Confidence

Run A Marathon With Confidence

ABOUT THE AUTHOR

Darryl Fry

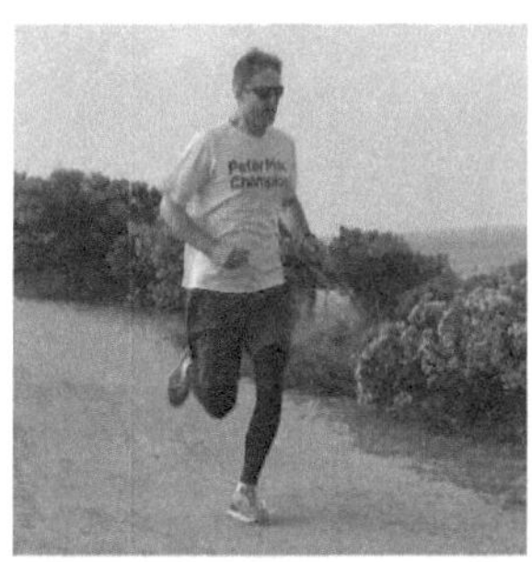

Darryl Fry is a former journalist who also has extensive experience in education, fitness and sports coaching.

After completing a journalism cadetship, he went on to major in Physical Education while obtaining a Bachelor of Education degree from Victoria University in Melbourne, Australia.

Darryl is also a qualified Health and Wellness Coach and Athletics Australia accredited Run Leader.

He has developed practical knowledge about health, fitness and living well through lifelong participation in physical activity.

Darryl has completed Sprint and Olympic Distance Triathlons and a variety of running events ranging in distance from 5km to the Marathon.

He lives in Hamilton, in the South West of Victoria, Australia.